UNLOCKING THE SECRET KEYS OF WEIGHT LOSS

The hidden keys to stubborn weight loss

ROSE JOHN JAMES

Table of content

Chapter 1

Weight loss and weight gain
You can lose fat and gain muscle

You lose muscle along with fat when you diet and lose weight rapidly. Consequently, you will acquire fat rather than muscle weight while you are yo-yo dieting and are gaining weight. This may eventually affect your capacity for walking, lifting objects, or climbing stairs.

Yo-yo dieting, or the rise and collapse of fad diets, is more typical than you may imagine, particularly with restrictive diets.

Check to see if you recognize this: To finally lose the weight you've wanted to, you worked really hard at the gym and followed a healthy diet for months... only to gain it all back as soon as you quit dieting. If this has occurred to you, it might seem like a hopeless cycle that never ends. The good news is that you're not alone in your difficulties and that you've already successfully shed some pounds.

Weight cycling, often known as yo-yo dieting, is a behavior characterized by a cycle of weight loss, weight gain, and then a new round of dieting. Yo-yo dieting prevents you from reaching your objectives because of the sometimes harsh highs and lows. Not to mention the potential long-term consequences for your health.
Fortunately, you can stop the pattern, lose your devotion to fad diets, and resume working toward your health objectives. How? Read on.

Why do people yo-yo diet?
You don't purposely yo-yo between diets. Your body reacts to unrealistic diets for physiological reasons. As you lose weight, the hormone leptin levels drop. Our bodies use leptin to alert us when we have enough energy (stored as fat) in reserve. We begin to

feel hungry after leptin levels drop sufficiently.

and if you abandon the tight diet, your chances of gaining it back increase.

The frequency of weight cycling?

There seems to be a new diet to try around every corner. Yo-yo dieting, or the rise and collapse of fad diets, is more typical than you may imagine, particularly with restrictive diets. 70% of the female participants in a March 2019 research from the Columbia University Irving Medical Center experienced weight cycling at least once. There were 485 women in the research, ranging in age from 20 to 76.

Weight changes are quite natural. Depending on what you eat, drink, and remove that day, your typical adult daily weight fluctuates between 3 and 4 pounds. It's not always necessary to cycle your weight dramatically. However, it often adheres to an unsustainable diet and falls outside of the body's natural parameters for weight loss and growth.

Why should you avoid yo-yo dieting?

You might gain fat while losing muscle.

You lose muscle along with fat when you diet and lose weight rapidly. Consequently, you will acquire fat rather than muscle weight while you are yo-yo dieting and are gaining weight. This may eventually affect your capacity for walking, lifting objects, or climbing stairs. With activity, such as weight training to guarantee muscular growth, this may be countered.

Weight cycling may raise body fat percentage, according to studies. The history of yo-yo dieting was linked to increased body fat in 11 out of 19 studies, according to an analysis of published literature. Weight cycling has also been associated with future weight gain, according to half of the research that was analyzed.

It poses a danger to your heart.
Your chance of acquiring heart disease rises as you acquire weight. The cycle of gaining and shedding weight follows a similar pattern. According to new research in the New England Journal of Medicine, the risk of heart disease increases as weight changes, and the bigger the swing in weight, the more likely it is.

Additionally, several researchers have looked at the connection between fluctuating weight and elevated blood pressure. According to earlier research, the effects of weight cycling on your blood pressure subside when enough time has passed. On this issue, however, not all research concur. According to more recent research, your body mass index will decide whether or not a history of weight cycling causes higher blood pressure. To get the whole picture, further study is required.

It might impact your emotional well-being.

Weight reduction is linked to many advantages for good mental health, including improved self-assurance, a feeling of accomplishment, and higher self-esteem. Unfortunately, there might also be drawbacks, particularly with yo-yo dieting. Weight fluctuations often are frustrating and may possibly exacerbate anxiety and sadness.

A 2020 research found that internalized weight stigma served as a mediator between a history of weight cycling and depressed symptoms. There was no discernible difference after controlling for gender, indicating that both men and women experience the same effects. Not everyone will experience this, much like the other risk factors on the list.

How to break the cycle of regaining weight

Dieting is challenging, and it's simpler than it should be to develop a weight cycling pattern. We don't want to give the impression that stopping the yo-yo dieting cycle is simple. It isn't. And keep in mind that being healthy does not require losing weight. However, if losing weight is your aim, this advice may be able to assist you take back control.

Review the diet you're following. Unsustainable diets are the foundation of yo-yo dieting. Any diets that cut out whole food groupings should be avoided. We need a cookie, a Coke, or a dish of spaghetti sometimes because we are humans. The freedom to choose what we eat and what we don't is most vital.

Consider the foods you are consuming. A good general rule of thumb is to attempt to steer clear of foods with high salt and sugar content. But don't deprive yourself of certain meals. One of the primary drawbacks of yo-yo dieting is that. Instead, make the decisions that are best for you by trying to strike a balance.

Exercise. Exercise is one of the key defenses against yo-yo diets. Keeping active can help you stick to your long-term weight reduction goal while maintaining a healthy weight. Exercise will also assist you in preventing the gradual loss of muscle mass. Just remember to take pauses and avoid overdoing it.

Be honest with yourself. On your trip, remember to check in with yourself. Are you sleeping well? What mood are you in? Have you altered how you feel about food? You can make sure you're healthy in all respects by periodically checking in on yourself.

Get help.

Yo-yo dieting has been connected to various types of disordered eating patterns, such as binge eating disorder. You can still receive assistance and work through your connection with food if meals and weight are unpleasant issues for you even if you don't have an eating disorder. Contact information for the National Eating Disorders Association hotline, a counselor, or your physician is available.

Here are the essential details.

Weight loss has a negative side, which is yo-yo dieting. And regrettably, a lot of individuals experience it. Keep in mind that losing weight does not always mean being healthy. Yo-yo dieting results from unsustainable, sometimes harmful diets that we are unable to follow. Even if you've been caught in the downward spiral of weight loss and gain, you may still break free of it.

Chapter 2

Do You Really Need 3 Meals a Day?

I've always eaten erratically, ever since I can remember. I hardly ever cook, and I have a nasty tendency of skipping meals until I'm so ravenously hungry that I'm nearly savage. I also snack like it's my job. An unusual triumph was eating three meals every day.

It's not just me. The percentage of persons who ate three meals a day dramatically decreased between the 1970s and 2010, according to the National Health and Nutrition Examination Survey (73% of men and 75% of women). Given that stress and burnout have just hit an all-time high, I'd hazard to say that those levels have decreased even more in the twelve years since that poll. Only nine out of 25 of my acquaintances, according to an informal survey we conducted this year, consume three square meals every day.

However, is it really important if you consume one, three, or six meals every day? Why is it so difficult if it's so important? In order to learn more, I conducted research and spoke with a nutrition specialist. Here are some positive changes in my personal eating habits.

Three meals each day: An explanation

The segmentation of your daily diet into three meals—breakfast, lunch, and dinner—hasn't always been the norm, and it still isn't in certain parts of the globe, despite the fact that we now take it for granted. Before industrialisation, Americans often ate only two substantial meals to prepare their bodies for rural, outdoor work, according to Amy Bentley of New York University's Center for Food History in an interview with The Atlantic. Two tiny, light meals were eaten in addition to one major meal in ancient Rome.

Our eating habits in the US are now often planned around our work or school schedules. Aside from cultural customs, there is no scientific justification for you to consume precisely three meals each day.

According to Marissa Kai Miluk, a registered dietitian nutritionist who focuses on preventing binge eating, "the number of meals in a day itself isn't essential." There is evidence on both sides of the spectrum on how often you "should" eat during the day, but each individual is unique.

There have been several studies conducted over the years that demonstrate both the advantages and drawbacks of eating more often. A few studies have also shown advantages to eating fewer, larger meals as well as, you guessed it, disadvantages.

Having said that, the advice to eat three meals a day wasn't given randomly. In a mathematical sense, it all boils down to this:

The typical adult needs 2,000 calories each day, yet there are only so many hours in the day. "Three meals a day is a general suggestion to support regular, appropriate energy consumption across all peer-reviewed studies and health practices," Miluk added. "I would not advocate eating fewer than three meals a day, since it would need a big intake in one sitting in order to fulfill basic requirements," she said. "Unless someone is really deficient in time or secure access to food.

However, the math may vary based on your own health requirements, schedule, and a variety of other, less quantitative considerations, such as, in my case, a love of munchies.

Consistency is more crucial than the total number of meals, according to Miluk. The unexpected consequences of skipping meals, waiting all day to eat, and other irregular eating habits may vary from elevated blood pressure to high or low blood sugar.

How can you determine if your eating habits are healthy?

Miluk said that typical indicators that you may need to review your eating habits and connection with food include frequent mood swings, hunger, irregular cravings, insatiable hunger, eating with a feeling of urgency, and binges.

But, at least for folks like myself, eating regular meals is so much more difficult than it sounds.

Why it's so difficult to eat three meals a day

The decision to deviate from the recommended three meals per day plan might occur from time to time. Even while it sounds ideal, it might be difficult to have a healthy breakfast, lunch, and supper every day. You can't always decide what meal alternatives are available or when you'll have time to sit down and eat. Hunger may also be impacted by stress and mental health.

Calling a spade a spade Eating takes effort. A meal requires time, effort, and money to prepare in addition to physical and mental exertion. When you have a million other things on your mind, even choosing what to eat might seem like an enormous challenge. And that's before you take into consideration diet culture, which elevates health and thinness to moral virtues, making mealtimes even more challenging and unpleasant. (If your only objective is weight reduction, meal time and frequency need a whole other kind of calculation.)

There is a lot of pressure to prepare all of your own meals with fresh, nutritious foods and to consume the "correct" amount and variety of meals. a tight budget. while working and looking after a family. Not as easy as it seems.

Sometimes it's more practical to simply grab for a snack rather than skipping all that. Over the years, fewer individuals have been eating three meals a day, but overall, calorie consumption has increased; the majority of those calories are now coming from snacks.

It might be rather simple to get wholesome meals that you don't have to prepare yourself in various nations. For instance, local foodways in Ghana and Mexico make it simple to stroll down the street and get a bundle of fresh local fruit or an inexpensive, completely cooked (and delicious) dinner made with local protein and produce. Not in many areas of the US, however.
There have been several studies conducted over the years that demonstrate both the advantages and drawbacks of eating more often. A few studies have also shown

advantages to eating fewer, larger meals as well as, you guessed it, disadvantages.

However, the math may vary based on your own health requirements, schedule, and a variety of other, less quantitative considerations, such as, in my case, a love of munchies.

Consistency is more crucial than the total number of meals, according to Miluk. The unexpected consequences of skipping meals, waiting all day to eat, and other irregular eating habits may vary from elevated blood pressure to high or low blood sugar.

How can you determine if your eating habits are healthy?

Miluk said that typical indicators that you may need to review your eating habits and connection with food include frequent mood swings, hunger, irregular cravings, insatiable hunger, eating with a feeling of urgency, and binges.

But, at least for folks like myself, eating regular meals is so much more difficult than it sounds.
Calling a spade a spade Eating takes effort. A meal requires time, effort, and money to prepare in addition to physical and mental exertion. When you have a million other things on your mind, even choosing what to eat might seem like an enormous challenge. And that's before you take into consideration diet culture, which elevates health and thinness to moral virtues, making mealtimes even more challenging and unpleasant. (If your only objective is weight reduction, meal time and frequency need a whole other kind of calculation.)

There is a lot of pressure to prepare all of your own meals with fresh, nutritious foods and to consume the "correct" amount and variety of meals. a tight budget. while working and looking after a family. Not as easy as it seems.

Sometimes it's more practical to simply grab for a snack rather than skipping all that. Over the years, fewer individuals have been eating three meals a day, but overall, calorie consumption has increased; the majority of those calories are now coming from snacks.

It might be rather simple to get wholesome meals that you don't have to prepare yourself in various nations. For instance, local foodways in Ghana and Mexico make it simple to stroll down the street and get a bundle of fresh local fruit or an inexpensive, completely cooked (and delicious) dinner made with local protein and produce. Not in many areas of the US, however.

However, the notion that you should prepare all of your meals at home yourself is just a new development. Only families with enough room for a home kitchen and the money to employ assistance could formerly afford to have daily meals prepared at home. Working-class residents of cities consumed prepared food from small eateries and street vendors. A treasured tradition in many cultures, both in the US and around the world, is communal eating.

Three meals a day isn't some magical number; it's just a benchmark to make sure you're consistently eating enough, which is very challenging in this country's modern lifestyle. What can you therefore do about it?

Three suggestions for consuming three meals

Priorities first: Recognize that having difficulty preparing three meals at home each day is not a personal failure. But to alleviate some of the annoyance, you don't necessarily have to wait for significant changes in society. Here are some pointers that worked for me and might work for you as well.

Revert to the fundamentals

Three meals a day is not a universal norm, as you are well aware of. But Miluk told me she normally counsels her clients to emphasize eating three meals a day first and foremost if they are having any difficulty eating regular meals at all.

She said, "When your body doesn't believe that food will always be accessible, it goes into fight-or-flight mode. A regular meal plan gives you a "strong basis" on which to reestablish your faith in your body and control your hunger.

It won't necessarily be easy sailing, however. I have a habit of accidentally missing lunch or putting off supper for far too long, and that hasn't changed. But having a specific objective in mind was quite beneficial. I discovered what it was like to enjoy life with constant energy instead of brain fog and hungriness every time I was able to have breakfast, lunch, and supper without any problems.

Use your best judgment.

I've tried many various strategies throughout the years to trick myself into eating my three meals. But until I ultimately gave up trying to constantly eat the "correct" things, the "right" manner, I can't really claim that I was able to achieve. Instead, I concentrated on what was practical and comfortable for me: how could I get the nutrients I needed while taking into consideration all the obstacles in my life?

You may be more inclined to really consume your three meals if you let go of any judgment about what they include. For me, it meant including meal shakes and a meal subscription into my daily schedule. Others may choose for grocery delivery, community assistance with meal preparation, canned or prepared meals, food trucks, or inexpensive, readily available produce (like bananas).

Everything changed for me when I decided to choose ease above health, even if it meant consuming foods I thought I "shouldn't" consume. I constantly remind myself that I'm worth the money and time it takes to take care of myself. I vow to taking care of myself in whatever manner I have to in spite of the fact that I forgive myself for living in a time and a society that make it difficult for me to nurture my body.

Be honest with yourself.

According to Miluk, after you've grown used to eating three meals a day, you can concentrate on learning to listen to your body's cues and utilizing the hunger-fullness scale to establish an eating pattern that suits you. This implies considering your dietary choices, health requirements and values, timetable, and accessibility. You may get assistance from a qualified nutritionist on your trip, but keep in mind that there is no universal recommendation for when or what to eat.

According to Miluk, the secret to determining when to eat is to tune out the outside environment and be completely honest with yourself.

She suggests asking the following inquiries to yourself in order to determine that:

- How do I feel compared to when I miss a meal when I routinely eat breakfast, lunch, and dinner?
- Can I go between meals and snacks without becoming hungry?
- Do I experience any changes in my ability to concentrate, energy level, or mood when I go for extended periods of time without a big meal or snack?
- Do I pay heed to my body's cues that indicate whether I am hungry or full?
- Is there anything about my hunger that stands out as unusual? Do I notice that my hunger varies

throughout the day or does it remain consistent?

For me, it turns out that eating three meals a day while working a 9 to 5 job is actually the most practical method to meet my daily requirements. That's simply what makes logical, given how frequently I become hungry and how much I prefer to eat at once. You may decide that eating two substantial meals each day, like farmers used to, or nibbling continuously is the key to living your best life. There's nothing wrong with those who call themselves "grazers," Miluk reassured me.

Chapter 3

Too much weight gain can lead to obesity

Obesity is a chronic, multifactorial condition that may result in excessive body fat and, sometimes, poor health. Of course, excess body fat itself is not an illness. However, an excessive amount of additional body fat might alter how your body works. These changes are gradual, have the potential to become worse over time, and may have a negative impact on health.

The good news is that by reducing part of your extra body fat, you may reduce your health risks. Your health may be significantly impacted by even little weight fluctuations. Every weight reduction strategy does not work for everyone. Most individuals have made many attempts to reduce weight. Additionally, maintaining a healthy weight is just as crucial as reducing weight initially.

Overeating and insufficient exercise are the two main contributors to obesity.

If you ingest a lot of calories, especially fat and sugar, but don't expand them via physical activity, the body will store a large portion of the excess calories as fat.

Calories

Calories are the units used to measure a food's energy content. To maintain a healthy weight, the typical physically active male requires around 2,500 calories per day, whereas the typical physically active woman needs about 2,000 calories per day.

This number of calories can seem excessive, but if you consume particular foods, it might be simple to attain. A big takeout hamburger, fries, and a milkshake, for instance, may add up to 1,500 calories in just one meal. Read our article on understanding calories for more details.

Another issue is that since so many people are inactive, a large portion of the calories they eat are converted to fat and stored in their bodies.

Bad diet

Obesity does not develop suddenly. It develops gradually over time as a result of poor dietary and lifestyle choices, such as consuming excessive amounts of processed or fast food that is high in fat and sugar, drinking excessive amounts of alcohol because it contains a lot of calories, and eating out frequently because you might be tempted to order an appetizer or dessert at a restaurant, which can be high in fat and sugar, and eating more than you need because you might be encouraged to do so.
If you have poor self-esteem or are unhappy, you could turn to comfort eating by consuming too many sugary beverages, such as soft drinks and fruit juice.
Eating disorders often run in families. When you're young, you could pick up unhealthy eating habits from your parents that you carry into adulthood.

Learn how reducing our intake of saturated fat and sugar impacts our health.

Absence of exercise

Another significant factor that contributes to obesity is a lack of physical exercise. Many individuals work professions that require them to spend the majority of the day seated at a desk. Additionally, they depend on their vehicles more than they do cycling or walking.

Most individuals seldom engage in regular exercise while they are relaxing instead preferring to watch TV, surf the internet, or play computer games.

The additional energy you consume is stored by the body as fat if you are not active enough to utilise the energy given by the food you eat.

Adults should engage in at least 150 minutes a week of moderate-intensity aerobic exercise, such as quick walking or cycling, according to the Department of Health and Social Care. This may be completed in tiny chunks over time and is not required to be done entirely at once. You may, for instance, work out for 30 minutes a day, five days a week.

You may need to exercise more than this if you are obese and attempting to reduce weight. Starting out gently and progressively increasing your weekly workout routine might be beneficial.

Learn more about the recommendations for adult physical exercise.

Genetics

Because "it runs in my family" or "it's in my genes," some individuals argue that there is no purpose in attempting to reduce weight.

Although there are a few uncommon hereditary disorders, such Prader-Willi syndrome, that may lead to obesity, most individuals can reduce weight without any problems.
It may be true that certain genetic characteristics you received from your parents, such as having a big appetite, make losing weight harder, but it's not impossible.

Obesity often has more to do with environmental variables, such bad eating practices picked up in childhood.

medical conditions
Substantial medical issues may sometimes cause weight gain. These consist of:
hypothyroidism, a condition in which your thyroid gland does not generate enough hormones
A uncommon condition called Cushing's syndrome results in the overproduction of steroid hormones.

However, if these problems are correctly identified and treated, they should lessen the difficulty of losing weight.

Weight gain is a side effect of various drugs, including some corticosteroids, diabetic and epilepsy treatments, as well as some drugs used to treat mental illness, such as antidepressants and schizophrenia meds.

Weight gain may sometimes occur as a result of quitting smoking.

It could be harder to lose weight if you have traits passed down from your parents, like a voracious appetite, but it's still achievable.

Obesity often has more to do with environmental variables, such bad eating practices picked up in childhood.

How does being obese impact my body?

Your body is impacted by obesity in various ways. Some of these consequences of having extra body fat are purely mechanical. For instance, it is easy to distinguish between more weight on your body and added strain on your joints and bones. More subdued impacts include blood chemistry changes that raise your risk for diabetes, heart disease, and stroke.

Some consequences still need to be better understood. For instance, obesity increases the chance of developing some malignancies. It exists, however we're not sure why. According to statistics, being obese raises your chance of dying young from any reason. Furthermore, research indicates that decreasing even a minor amount of weight (5% to 10%) might greatly reduce these chances.

metabolic adjustments

Your metabolism is the process through which calories are transformed into energy to power various bodily processes. Your body turns excess calories into lipids and stores them in your adipose tissue when there are more calories than it can consume (body fat). The size of the fat cells themselves increases when there is no longer any tissue in which to store lipids. Hormones and other substances that cause inflammation are secreted by enlarged fat cells.

The impacts of chronic inflammation on health are many. It influences your metabolism by causing insulin resistance, among other things. This indicates that your body can no longer effectively decrease blood sugar and cholesterol levels with the help of insulin (sugars and fats in your blood). Excessive blood pressure is also a result of high blood sugar and blood lipids (cholesterol and triglycerides).

The term "metabolic syndrome" refers to these risk factors taken together. They are included because they all often reinforce one another. Additionally, they encourage continued weight gain and make it more difficult to reduce weight and maintain weight reduction. Metabolic syndrome is a frequent contributor to obesity and numerous disorders that are associated to it, such as:

diabetes type 2. Obesity especially increases the risk of Type 2 diabetes by seven and twelve times, respectively, depending on the gender allocated at birth. For every extra point on the BMI scale, the risk rises by 20%. It also becomes smaller as you lose weight.
cardiovascular conditions Heart disease risk factors include high blood pressure, high cholesterol, high blood sugar, and inflammation. These conditions include coronary artery disease, congestive heart failure, heart attack, and stroke. Your BMI goes hand in hand with an increase in these hazards. The biggest cause of avoidable mortality globally and in the United States is cardiovascular disease.
fat in the liver. Your liver, which is in charge of filtering your blood, receives extra lipids

that are circulating in your blood. The accumulation of extra fat in your liver may cause chronic liver inflammation (hepatitis) and long-term liver damage (cirrhosis).
kidney illness Among the most frequent causes of chronic kidney disease are high blood pressure, diabetes, and liver disease.
Gallstones. Higher blood cholesterol levels may result in gallstones and other possible gallbladder problems by causing cholesterol to build up in your gallbladder.

Direct results

The respiratory system's organs may get crowded by excess body fat, and your musculoskeletal system may experience tension and pressure. Asthma is a result of this.
Apneic sleep.
the syndrome of obesity hypoventilation.
Osteoarthritis.
back ache
Gout.

The American Centers for Disease Control and Prevention report that 1 in 3 obese persons also have arthritis. According to studies, the likelihood of developing knee arthritis rises by 36% for every 5 kg you acquire. The good news is that a 10% weight reduction combined with exercise may considerably lessen discomfort from arthritis and enhance your quality of life.

immediate consequences
Additionally, obesity has indirect links to:

Memory and cognition, including an increased risk of dementia and Alzheimer's disease.
problems during pregnancy and female infertility.
depression and mental health issues.
Esophageal, pancreatic, colorectal, breast, uterine, and ovarian malignancies are only a few examples.

How is overweight managed?

Your unique treatment plan will be based on your overall health profile. Your healthcare professional will start by addressing your most pressing health issues before moving on to a longer-term weight reduction strategy. They may sometimes suggest short modifications that have an instant effect, like changing your prescription. The overall course of therapy will be more slow and likely entail several variables. Finding the treatments that are most effective for you may need some trial and error since everyone is unique. Studies have consistently demonstrated that the most effective methods for assisting individuals to lose weight and keep it off are aggressive, team-based programs with regular, one-on-one contact between your physician and you.

Your therapy program may consist of:

Diet modifications

You alone will know what dietary adjustments you need to make to reduce weight. Cutting down on snacks between meals or portion sizes may be beneficial for some individuals. Others may be more concerned with altering what they eat than how much. Eating more vegetables is advantageous for almost everyone. Fruits, vegetables, whole grains, and legumes often have greater fiber and micronutrient contents than they do fat. You might feel fuller and more pleased after consuming fewer calories because they are more nutrient-dense.

Heightened activity

Everyone is aware of the need for both food and exercise for weight reduction and weight maintenance. But working out doesn't always need a gym membership. One of the most effective forms of exercise for losing weight is just walking at a moderate speed. Five days a week, for only

30 minutes, is what healthcare professionals advise. A regular stroll before or after work, at lunch, or at other times may really make a difference.

Psychological treatments

Your weight reduction journey may be assisted by counseling, support groups, and techniques like cognitive behavioral therapy. Your brain may be rewired to encourage beneficial changes using these techniques. They may also assist you in controlling stress and addressing any emotional or psychological issues that could be hindering your progress. We are impacted by our weight and attempts to lose it on many different levels, so having support on both a psychological and practical level may be beneficial.

Medication

Your doctor could suggest using some drugs in addition to other therapies. While they don't provide a complete solution, medications might assist approach weight reduction from a different perspective. For instance, medications that suppress your appetite might block some of the brain circuits that control your hunger. This could be a little piece of the jigsaw for some, but it might be a larger one for others.

FDA-approved medications often used to treat obesity include:

Reduces the absorption of fat from your intestines with orlistat (Xenical®, Alli®).
Reduces appetite: Phentermine (Adipex-P, Lomaira, Suprenza). It may be used for three months straight.
The stimulant benzphetamine (Didrex®, Regimex®) reduces appetite.
Reduces appetite: Diethylpropion (Depletite #2®, Radtue®, Tenuate®).
Reduces appetite: Phendimetrazine (Bontril®, Melfiat®).
Intake of food and desires may be decreased with bupropion-naltrexone (Contrave®).

Liraglutide (Saxenda®): Sluggish digestion and decreases hunger.
Wegov Semaglutide ® 's (suppresses appetite).
Plenty® (cellulose and citric acid): Gives you a full feeling.
Lisdexamfetamine dimesylate (Vyvanse®): Aids in managing binge eating disorder symptoms.
Reduces Appetite. Phentermine-topiramate (Qsymia®).
SGLT2 inhibitors combined with glucagon-like receptor agonists.

Surgery to lose weight

If you have been classified as having class III obesity, you may be a candidate for bariatric surgery. Surgery is a drastic yet very efficient way to lose considerable amounts of weight over the long term. Instead of merely affecting your thinking or behaviors, it also alters your biology. Your digestive tract is affected in some manner by every bariatric surgery treatment. They limit how many calories you can take in and assimilate. Additionally, they alter digestive system hormones that influence your metabolism and appetite.

Procedures used in bariatric surgery include:

stomach sleeve (sleeve gastrectomy).
stomach band (LAP band).
stomach bypass (Roux-en-Y).
the duodenal switch

How can I avoid being obese?

It is simpler to prevent obesity than to cure it once it has set in. Your body will take it as your new baseline weight after it has established a new high "set point." Despite your aspirations to lose weight, your body attempts to control your hunger signals and energy expenditure in order to maintain the same body mass.

You may want to act sooner rather than later to intervene if you've detected a trend of recent weight increase in yourself or your kid, or if you have a family history of obesity. You may avoid future obesity and weight loss issues by taking an honest look at your behaviors and making realistic adjustments now.

For instance:

Make a modest decision. Do you often use a calorie-dense sweet drink as a "pick-me-up" or daily habit? Think about replacing it. Up to 10 additional pounds might be gained in a year with only 150 more calories each day. That is equivalent to two double-stuffed Oreo cookies or a snack-size bag of potato chips.
Include a quick activity. Instead, think about what you might do to burn an additional 150 calories every day. Take the dog for a 35-minute brisk walk, for instance, or spend

25 minutes hiking or using an elliptical machine.

Shopping on purpose Maintain a healthy food supply in your house and save desserts and other pleasures for special occasions when you go out. In contrast to manufactured snacks and sweets, which cause your blood sugar to rise and fall, whole foods are richer in fiber and lower on the glycemic index.

Promote general well-being. Reduce your screen time and take a stroll outdoors instead. To keep your hormone levels in line, control your stress and make an effort to get enough sleep. Place more emphasis on wholesome activities and beneficial improvements than on how your actions affect your weight.

Chapter 4

Reduce Belly Fat and Rev up Sluggish Metabolism

More than just an annoyance that makes your clothing feel snug is belly fat.

It causes considerable injury.

Visceral fat, one form of belly fat, is a significant risk factor for type 2 diabetes, heart disease, and other illnesses (1Trusted Source).

Body mass index (BMI) is widely used in the medical field to categorize weight and determine the likelihood of developing metabolic diseases.

This is false, however, since those with extra abdominal fat are at a higher risk even if they seem to be slender (2 Trusted Source).

There are a few things you may do to lose extra abdominal fat even though it might be challenging to lose fat from this region.

Here are some efficient weight-loss strategies supported by research.

1. Consume a lot of soluble fiber

The gel that is created when soluble fiber absorbs water aids in slowing down the passage of food through your digestive tract. According to studies, this sort of fiber aids in weight reduction by making you feel full, which causes you to eat less naturally. Additionally, it can decrease the quantity of calories your body takes in from meals (3Trusted Source, 4Trusted Source, 5Trusted Source).

Soluble fiber may also aid in the battle against abdominal obesity.

In a 5-year observational study of over 1,100 people, it was shown that belly fat accumulation reduced by 3.7% for every 10-gram increase in soluble fiber consumption (6Trusted Source).

Make an effort to eat meals rich in fiber each day. The following are excellent sources of soluble fiber:

hemp seeds
noodles in shirataki
Belgian spuds
avocados\legumes
blackberries

SUMMARY
You could lose weight by consuming more soluble fiber, which also makes you feel fuller while consuming less calories. In your diet plan for losing weight, try to consume a lot of foods rich in fiber.

2.Avoid trans-fat-containing foods.
By injecting hydrogen into unsaturated fats like soybean oil, trans fats are produced.
Although certain margarines and spreads still include them, many food manufacturers have discontinued using them. They are also often added to packaged goods.
In observational and animal research, these lipids have been linked to inflammation, heart disease, insulin resistance, and belly

fat growth (7Trusted Source, 8Trusted Source, 9Trusted Source).

In a 6-year research, it was shown that monkeys that consumed more trans fat developed 33% more belly fat than those who consumed more monounsaturated fat (10 Trusted Source).

Read ingredient labels carefully and steer clear of goods that contain trans fats to aid in belly fat reduction and safeguard your health. Partially hydrogenated fats are often used to describe them.

A high trans fat diet has been related in certain studies to an increase in belly fat growth. Regardless of whether you're attempting to lose weight, it's a good idea to restrict your consumption of trans fat.

3. Restrict your alcohol consumption.

Alcohol may be beneficial to your health in moderation, but excessive use can be quite dangerous.

According to research, drinking too much alcohol may also contribute to belly fat accumulation.

Heavy drinking is associated with a considerably higher risk of central obesity, or excess fat accumulation around the waist, according to observational research (11Trusted Source, 12Trusted Source).

Reducing your alcohol consumption may aid in weight loss. While you don't have to stop entirely, cutting down on how much you consume each day might be beneficial.

More than 2,000 participants participated in one research on alcohol usage.

According to the findings, people who regularly drank alcohol but only had one or fewer drinks on average per day had less belly fat than those who drank less often but more frequently on the days they did (12 Trusted Source).

SUMMARY

An increase in abdominal fat has been linked to excessive alcohol use. If you want to lose weight, think about consuming alcohol in moderation or not at all.

4. Consume a lot of protein.

A crucial nutrient for controlling weight is protein.

A high protein diet boosts the production of the hormone PYY that promotes fullness and suppresses hunger.

Additionally, protein increases metabolism and aids in maintaining muscle mass when dieting (13 Trusted Source, 14 Trusted Source, 15 Trusted Source).

Numerous observational studies reveal that those who consume more protein have lower rates of belly fat than those who consume less protein (16 Trusted Source, 17Trusted Source, 18Trusted Source).

At each meal, be sure to incorporate a quality protein source, such as:

Meat, fish, eggs, milk, whey protein, and legumes

SUMMARY

If you're aiming to lose weight around your waist, high protein diets like fish, lean meat, and beans are recommended.

5. Lessen your degree of tension

By causing the adrenal glands to generate cortisol, often known as the stress hormone, stress might cause you to put on belly fat.

According to studies, increased cortisol levels promote hunger and belly fat accumulation (19 Trusted Source, 20Trusted Source).

Additionally, women with big waists tend to respond to stress by producing more cortisol. Increased cortisol contributes to further belly fat growth (21Trusted Source).

Participate in enjoyable stress-relieving hobbies to aid in abdominal fat reduction. Yoga and meditation are both useful techniques.

SUMMARY

Your waistline may acquire weight as a result of stress. If you're attempting to reduce weight, one of your top objectives should be minimizing stress.

6. Limit your intake of sugary foods.

Sugar-added foods are unhealthy for your health. Consuming an excessive amount of these foods might result in weight gain.

According to studies, adding sugar has particularly detrimental impacts on metabolic health (3Trusted Source).

Numerous studies have shown that too much sugar, mostly because of the high fructose content, may cause fat to accumulate around your liver and belly (6).

Half of sugar is fructose and half is glucose. The liver becomes overwhelmed with fructose when you consume a lot of added sugar and is compelled to convert it to fat (4Trusted Source, 5).

Some people think that this is the primary mechanism behind sugar's detrimental impacts on health. It raises liver and belly fat, which causes insulin resistance and a number of metabolic issues (7Trusted Source).

In this aspect, liquid sugar is worse. Drinking sugar-sweetened drinks causes you to consume more calories overall because the brain doesn't seem to register liquid calories in the same way as solid calories (8 Trusted Source, 9Trusted Source).

According to a research, children's risk of becoming obese increased by 60% with every extra daily serving of sugar-sweetened drinks (10).

Reduce your intake of sugar and think about cutting out all sugar-sweetened beverages. This includes drinks with added sugar, sugary sodas, fruit juices, and other sports drinks with a lot of added sugar.

Make sure items don't contain refined sugars by reading the labels. Even meals that are promoted as healthy might have large sugar content.

Remember that none of this applies to entire fruit, which are very nutritious and contain a lot of fiber, which counteracts the bad effects of fructose.

SYNOPSIS A lot of people's excessive sugar consumption contributes significantly to weight gain. Eat less confectionery and processed food that has extra sugar.

7. Exercise aerobically (cardio)

Cardiovascular exercise (cardio) is a great strategy to burn calories and enhance your health.

It's also one of the best exercises for decreasing abdominal fat, according to studies. Results on whether moderate or vigorous exercise is better for you, nevertheless, are conflicting (27 Trusted Source, 28Trusted Source, 29Trusted Source).

In any case, the frequency and length of your workout regimen are more crucial than the level of difficulty.

According to one research, postmenopausal women who engaged in aerobic activity for

300 minutes a week shed more fat overall than those who exercised for 150 minutes a week (30Trusted Source).

SUMMARY
Exercise that is aerobic is a good way to lose weight. According to studies, it's especially helpful in reducing waist size.

8. Reduce your intake of carbohydrates, particularly processed ones.

You may lose a lot of fat, particularly belly fat, by cutting down on your carb consumption.

Overweight individuals, those at risk for type 2 diabetes, and women with polycystic ovary syndrome (PCOS) who follow diets with less than 50 grams of carbohydrates per day lose belly fat (31 Trusted Source, 32Trusted Source, 33Trusted Source).

You do not need to adhere to a rigorous low-carb diet. According to several studies, merely substituting unprocessed starchy carbohydrates for refined carbohydrates will enhance metabolic health and decrease belly fat (34 Trusted Source, 35Trusted Source).

According to the renowned Framingham Heart Study, persons who eat the most whole grains were 17% less likely than those who ingested the most refined grains to develop extra belly fat (36 Trusted Source).

SUMMARY

Excessive abdominal fat is linked to a large consumption of refined carbohydrates. Consider lowering your carb consumption or substituting healthy carb sources like whole grains, legumes, or vegetables for refined carbohydrates in your diet.

9. Exercise with resistance (lift weights)

For the purpose of maintaining and growing muscular mass, resistance training—also referred to as weightlifting or strength training—is crucial.

Resistance exercise may also help with belly fat reduction, according to research including persons with prediabetes, type 2 diabetes, and fatty liver disease (37 Trusted Source, 38Trusted Source).

In fact, a study of overweight teens found that the most effective way to reduce visceral fat was to combine strength training with aerobic activity (39 Trusted Source).

Asking assistance from a licensed personal trainer is a smart move if you decide to start weightlifting.

SYNOPSIS Strength training may be a crucial component of a weight reduction plan and may help decrease abdominal fat. Studies indicate that when combined with aerobic activity, it is considerably more beneficial.

10. Steer clear of drinks with added sugar.

Liquid fructose, which is abundant in drinks with added sugar and might cause you to build belly fat,
According to studies, drinking sugary beverages causes the liver to store more fat. One 10-week research discovered that those who drank high-fructose drinks significantly increased their belly fat (40 Trusted Source, 41Trusted Source, 42Trusted Source).
Drinks with added sugar seem to be worse than meals with added sugar.
You're prone to overeat calories later on and store them as fat since your brain doesn't handle liquid calories the same way it processes solid ones (43Trusted Source, 44Trusted Source).
It's advisable to entirely avoid sugar-sweetened drinks like soda punch and sweet tea if you want to decrease abdominal fat.
alcohol mixers with added sugar

SUMMARY

If you're attempting to lose some weight, it's crucial to refrain from consuming any liquid forms of sugar, including drinks with added sugar.

11. Get plenty of quality sleep

Weight loss is only one of the many areas of health that sleep affects. People who don't get enough sleep tend to accumulate extra weight, which may include belly fat, according to studies (45 Trusted Source, 46Trusted Source).

According to a 16-year research involving more than 68,000 women, those who slept for fewer than 5 hours a night had a much higher risk of gaining weight than those who slept for 7 hours or more (47 Trusted Source).

Excess visceral fat has also been connected to the disease known as sleep apnea, which causes breathing to halt periodically during the night (48Trusted Source).

Make sure you get enough good sleep in addition to obtaining at least 7 hours each night.

Speak with a doctor and be treated if you think you could have sleep apnea or another kind of sleep disturbance.

SUMMARY

Lack of sleep is associated with a higher risk of gaining weight. If you want to reduce weight and become healthier, one of your top concerns should be getting enough good sleep.

12. Monitor your diet and exercise.

There are several ways to reduce your weight and belly fat, but the most important is to consume less calories than your body requires to maintain your weight (49 Trusted Source).

You may keep track of your calorie consumption by keeping a food journal or by utilizing an app or online meal tracker. It has been shown that using this method

would help you lose weight (50Trusted Source, 51Trusted Source).
Additionally, food-tracking apps enable you to know how much protein, carbohydrates, fiber, and micronutrients you are consuming. Many also let you keep track of your physical activities and workouts.
This article lists five free tools for tracking calorie and nutrient consumption.

SUMMARY
Keeping note of what you eat is usually a smart idea as basic weight reduction advice. The two most common methods for doing this are keeping a meal journal or utilizing an online food tracker.

13.consume fatty fish once a week.
Fish with fat are very healthy.
They are abundant in high-quality protein and disease-preventing omega-3 fatty acids (52 Trusted Source, 53Trusted Source).

According to some studies, these omega-3 fatty acids may also aid in the reduction of visceral fat.

Supplementing with fish oil may considerably decrease liver and abdominal fat, according to studies in both adults and children with fatty liver disease (54 Trusted Source, 55Trusted Source, 56Trusted Source).

Try to eat two to three portions of fatty fish per week. Good options include of:

salmon\herring\sardines\mackerel\anchovies

14.Consume probiotic-rich meals or supplements.

Bacteria known as probiotics are present in several meals and supplements. They provide several health advantages, including strengthening the immune system and promoting gastrointestinal health (64 Trusted Source).

Researchers have discovered that several bacterial species play a part in controlling weight and that achieving the appropriate balance may aid in weight loss, including the reduction of belly fat.

Members of the Lactobacillus family, particularly Lactobacillus gasseri, Lactobacillus fermentum, and Lactobacillus amylovorus, have been found to decrease belly fat (65Trusted Source, 66, 67Trusted Source, 68Trusted Source).

Make sure the probiotic supplement you choose has one or more of these bacterial strains since probiotic supplements generally include many different kinds of bacteria.

SUMMARY

A healthy digestive system may be supported by taking probiotic supplements. Additionally, studies indicate that healthy gut flora may support weight reduction.

15. Examine sporadic fasting

As a weight reduction strategy, intermittent fasting has lately gained a lot of popularity.

It is a schedule of eating that alternates between eating and fasting times (69Trusted Source).

One well-liked technique is once or twice weekly 24-hour fasts. Another involves consuming all of your meals in eight hours after a 16-hour fast each day.

In a review of research on alternate-day and intermittent fasting, patients saw a 4-7% reduction in abdominal fat over the course of 6–24 weeks (70).

There is some evidence to suggest that fasting in general, including intermittent fasting, may not be as helpful for women as it is for males.

Even while certain modified forms of intermittent fasting seem to be preferable, you should quit fasting right once if you encounter any side effects.

SUMMARY

An eating pattern known as intermittent fasting alternates between eating and fasting times. It may be one of the best methods to decrease weight and abdominal fat, according to studies.

16. Sip some green tea

An especially healthful beverage is green tea.

Epigallocatechin gallate (EGCG), an antioxidant, and caffeine are both present, and they both seem to increase metabolism (71 Trusted Source, 72Trusted Source).

Catechins like EGCG, which may aid in belly fat loss, have been the subject of several research. When green tea and exercise are combined, the impact can be enhanced (73 Trusted Source, 74, 75 Trusted Source).

Regular use of green tea has been associated with weight reduction, while it is likely less effective when taken alone and works best when paired with physical activity.

The conclusion

There are no quick fixes for getting rid of tummy fat.

It always takes work, dedication, and persistence on your part to lose weight.

You will undoubtedly reduce the excess weight around your waist if you are successful in implementing some or all of the lifestyle objectives and tactics outlined in this article.

Chapter 5

Consistency and diligence are required for a successful outcome.

Consistency is key, and because hard effort pays off in the long run, brilliance will follow. I've discovered from experience that you can achieve greater success if you put in more effort, more time, and more consistency.

One of the main things that contributes to achievement and success is consistency.

For you to succeed and reach your objectives, consistency must be combined with self-discipline.

Your muscular strength and endurance may both increase with regular exercise. Exercise helps your circulatory system function more effectively and distributes oxygen and nutrients to your tissues. Additionally, you have greater energy to do everyday tasks as your heart and lung health improves.

Set a sensible objective for your body type.

- Exercise your heart and your muscles.
- Make sure you're doing your workouts thoroughly and properly.
- Make sure you are always challenged throughout your exercises.
- Be dependable and forgiving.
- Keep your relaxation days.
- Improve your diet.
- Consider a change in lifestyle.

Additionally, if you workout often, you will eventually get even greater fitness advantages. In 3 to 4 months, you may significantly remodel your health and fitness. "At 6 to 8 weeks, you can clearly detect some improvements," stated Logie. Results for each strength take roughly the same time.

www.ingramcontent.com/pod-product-compliance
Lightning Source LLC
LaVergne TN
LVHW050340160826
845677LV00014B/3711

* 9 7 9 8 8 4 8 8 2 5 8 4 8 *